French Secrets about Beauty & Fashion

La Vie en Rose

"Like The French" Series, Book 3

Lesleigh Kivedo

French Secrets about Beauty & Fashion

Copyright © 2019

All rights reserved. This book or any portion thereof may not be reproduced or used in any manner whatsoever without the express written permission of the publisher except for the use of brief quotations in a book review.

ISBN: 9781670350718

Warning and Disclaimer

Every effort has been made to make this book as accurate as possible. However, no warranty or fitness is implied. The information provided is on an "as-is" basis. The author and the publisher shall have no liability or responsibility to any person or entity with respect to any loss or damages that arise from the information in this book.

Publisher Contact

Skinny Bottle Publishing
books@skinnybottle.com

Lesleigh Kivedo:

A self-confessed Francophile at heart, Lesleigh Kivedo has been writing about fashion, beauty, health and travel for over 10 years. Starting her career as an editorial intern at *Marie Claire* magazine (yes, like Anne Hathaway in *The Devil Wears Prada*), she then found her fashion feet as a features writer for *Cosmopolitan* magazine in South Africa. Her travels have since taken her to Montreal, Amsterdam, Bali, Dubai and, of course, her beloved Paris. These days, when not re-watching *Paris Je T'aime*, she continues with her passion for writing as a lifestyle journalist, covering everything from the up-and-coming fashion tendencies to the latest Kimye baby.

LIKE THE FRENCH 1

BEAUTY 3

    A FACIAL IS NOT A LUXURY. IT'S A WAY OF LIFE. 5

    IN SKINCARE, THE GENTLER, THE BETTER 5

    WRINKLES ARE NOT THE END OF THE WORLD. IN FACT, THEY ADD CHARACTER. 6

    LEARN TO GIVE A PROPER MASSAGE 8

    PATIENCE IS A VIRTUE 8

    BUT SOMETIMES THE FRENCH WAY IS NOT ALWAYS BETTER… 9

    SUNTANNING WITHOUT SPF 9

    SMOKING TO A FAULT 9

Time 11

Water 15

    MICELLAR WATER 16

    THERMAL WATER FACE MIST 17

    FLORAL WATER 18

    MARINE MIST 18

    BEAUTY MIST 19

The Classics 20

From the mouths of bébés 26

    WE JUST WANT TO LOOK FRESHER, BUT THAT'S IT 26

    IT'S ALL ABOUT BALANCE 26

    YOU LOOK BETTER WITHOUT MAKEUP 27

    THREE STEPS ARE ALL YOU NEED 27

    THE ONE THING YOU CAN FAKE: FRECKLES 27

    THE FRENCH MANICURE IS NOT FRENCH 28

    TOUSLED HAIR IS YOUR SECRET WEAPON 28

    IT'S ALL IN THE LINING 28

    PERFECT YOUR POUT 29

    MIX YOUR MASCARA.. 29

Hair 30

    THE BEDHEAD... 30

    BALAYAGE COLOR 32

    FRENCH BANGS 33

Perfume.. 35

    YOUR FRAGRANCE DEFINES YOU, SO CHOOSE WISELY 36

    BUT YOUR FRAGRANCE SHOULD ALSO GROW WITH YOU................. 36

    DISCRETION IS KEY 37

    REMEMBER THE FRAGRANCE ETIQUETTE.. 38

Smell like a Frenchie... 39

    The First Fragrance: Cacharel Anaïs Anaïs 39

    The Modern Parisian Scent: Chanel Coco Mademoiselle 40

    The Ultimate Classic: Chanel No. 5 40

    The Scent of Sophistication: Guerlain Shalimar 40

    FASHION 41

    MOST IMPORTANTLY, WEAR WHAT FEELS RIGHT 41

    IT'S A BOY/GIRL THING... 43

    UNKEMPT GLAMOUR 45

    EMBRACE THE CLASSICS... 47

    YOUR COMFORT MATTERS 49

    VARIETY IS OKAY TOO 51

    GLAMOUR IS IN THE UNEXPECTED 53

A French Sense 55

    ALL BLACK EVERYTHING 56

    A CLASH OF PRIMARY COLORS 57

    MODERN MEETS VINTAGE 59

    FAUX FUR AND STILETTOS.. 59

SLIGHTLY OVERSIZED DOES THE TRICK	62
Dressing	*64*
COMBINE CLASSIC WHITE WITH DIAMONDS	64
DON'T BE AFRAID OF A LITTLE SPARKLE	66
WORK WITH YOUR PROPORTIONS	68
MAKE COLOR WORK FOR YOU	70
ADORN YOURSELF IN BLACK FRENCH LACE	72
NAVY BLUE – THE SOFTER CHOICE	74
FEMININITY RULES	76
CUTE AND STILL SEXY	77
TEA LENGTH FOR UNDERSTATED GLAMOUR	79
IT'S OKAY TO BE A LITTLE DRAMATIC	80
French Women	*82*
JEANNE DAMAS	82
ALMA JODOROWSKY	83
FANNY PÉCHIODAT	83
CAMILLE ROWE	84
MORGANE SEZALORY	84
FATOU N'DIAYE	85
ADÈLE EXARCHOPOULOS	85
ANNE-LAURE MAIS or ADENORAH	86
LOUISE FOLLAIN	86
DENNI ELIAS	87
One Last Thing	**89**

LIKE THE FRENCH

Which nation in the world has the most stylish women? If your immediate answer was "France, obviously"… welcome. You've joined the ranks of an ever-growing fascination with all things français.

And you're not alone. There has been an overwhelming interest in Gallic style over the past decade, with every self-respecting women's interest blog and magazine website devoting a regular section to French Girl Style.

"I think when you live in an old country like France, and you've always been surrounded by architecture and buildings, you're used to learning what beauty is," explains Caroline de Maigret, speaking to Harper's Bazaar magazine about the inspiration behind her style tome How to Be Parisian Wherever You Are: Love, Style, and Bad Habits. "And you have a respect for fabrics and art, and handmade things and quality, and you know fashion—couture was more or less born in Paris. So we do have this, and because it's not a culture of showing off, we're completely fine about wearing the same jacket every day. It's more about wearing the right jacket or having the right face that fits you, that you want to show people the right makeup. It's more about finding who you are."

And so, in the spirit of infusing our own lives with some of their ethereal style and grace, we've compiled your go-to guide on French beauty and fashion. Ready? C'est parti!

BEAUTY

Être bien dans sa peau
(to be happy in one's skin)

What is the true essence of je ne sais quoi? You know, that mystifying, enigmatic quality that makes French women so unequivocally chic? Is it something all Gallic women are naturally born with? They'd sure like you to think so. "I think the concept—it's not a concept, because it's instinctive—but I think the idea is that the French woman doesn't want to show that she took some time taking care of herself. She wants you to think that she has better things to do, although she spends as much time [as you do]," says de Maigret. "She wants to be loved for her personality rather than for her décolletage, for her appeal. She wants to look beautiful, she wants you to think that she looks beautiful, but at the end of a dinner she wants someone to say, 'wow, it was a great conversation, we had a lot of fun,' rather than, 'oh she looks good!'"

So is there really such a vast difference between the French and women from elsewhere in the world? Online beauty store Escentual.com conducted a survey where they asked the readers to guess the age of French actress

Marion Cotillard. Of those who responded, the majority reckoned that the La Vie En Rose star was 35 years old. The truth? At the time of the survey, Cotillard was 41 – a whopping six years older. Vanessa Paradis similarly was thought to be seven years younger – 37 years old instead of her actual 44. What the survey also found was that, for every decade, French women were thought to look 1.35 years younger than their British counterparts.

So what's the big difference? Well, it may all start with their mothers, in more ways than one. In France, it is customary for mothers to start taking their daughters for regular facials at their own aesthetician starting from their 13th birthdays. So says Laetitia Labassee, the educational director at French skincare brand Darphin.

Where does that leave the rest of us; those born without aesthetically-inclined parents? To start with, it may be as simple as a shift in our mindset. Start thinking like the French do. The mode de vie française relies heavily on the concept of restoring nature's balance. That means spending as much (if not more) time on rest and relaxation as you do on your work and career life. Simple pleasures in life take precedent – long, languid meals with friends and family savoring the best quality food, for example. Similarly, the onus on taking care of oneself is placed high on the list of priorities. A Frenchwoman aims to balance the stress of her daily life with equal parts of restorative me-time.

In today's fast-paced, career-driven world, this type of pampering can seem almost self-indulgent and narcissistic. Not so in France. Celebrity skincare expert and aesthetician Renée Rouleau admires this natural approach to beauty. She may be based in the United States but regularly takes trips to France to catch up on the latest research and advances in skincare. She shares with us her top skincare commandments, the French way.

A FACIAL IS NOT A LUXURY. IT'S A WAY OF LIFE.

"My mum took me and my sister to a dermatologist, just once, when we were teenagers - to teach us the basics of what to do to take care of our skin. It's obviously a time when skin can become a problem, so he just gave us advice for the years ahead," French actress Clémence Poésy told British Vogue. And it makes sense. Teenage skin has its own set of concerns – hormonal, cystic acne and oiliness to name just a few.

For the majority of French women, it doesn't stop there. "Prevention is the key to their beautiful skin," says Rouleau. French women diligently schedule standing appointments with their aestheticians every month (yes, every French woman has one). "Many American women wait until years later to get serious about their skin in hopes of erasing the skin sins of their past," she says. By visiting an expert regularly and developing a longstanding relationship, your aesthetician will get to know your skin thoroughly. Best of all, so will you. You will learn precisely which products are catered to your skin's particular needs. This is definitely not the same service you would receive from a beauty consultant at a department store.

IN SKINCARE, THE GENTLER, THE BETTER

This is probably where French skincare differs the most from the American variety. In France, any chemicals are regarded with extreme skepticism. Generally, if there is a natural ingredient that can address a certain skincare issue, that substance will always be preferred over any chemical, synthetic substitute. The same goes for any harsh, abrasive treatments.

Microdermabrasion, a beauty trend that has really caught on in the US over the past few years, along with harsh exfoliants, lasers, and chemical peels are simply not tolerated in France. "Many French estheticians never embraced microdermabrasion technology because it seemed too harsh on the skin and French aestheticians are all about being gentle," says Rouleau. "Even AHA's (Alpha Hydroxy Acids) aren't as popular in France as they are here in the U.S." One explanation for this phenomenon might just be the simple fact that French women have spent their entire lives looking after their skin. "The prevention they have taken with their skin allows them to not have to seek these treatments to "fix" the damage done on the skin. "

WRINKLES ARE NOT THE END OF THE WORLD. IN FACT, THEY ADD CHARACTER.

Mieux vaut prévenir que guérir. If French beauty could be summed up in a single phrase, this one would most likely be it. It translates into English as "It's better to prevent than to heal" and relates as much to health, diet, and fitness as it does to beauty.

It's very rare to find a French woman who has had cosmetic surgery. As Rouleau explains: "A French woman told me once, 'Getting cosmetic procedures is a tell-tale sign of insecurity. Accept who you are, and work with what you have'." The French philosophy is to make the most of what you have. They will simply not change any part of themselves to meet an unnatural idea of beauty. "They take a very holistic approach and embrace their natural beauty. Self-acceptance is very strong for the women of France," says Rouleau.

One small lifestyle change you can make to keep wrinkles at bay – dermatologist-approved – is learning to sleep on your back. Think of your typical nighttime sleeping position. Does it involve your face being squashed into the pillow? Chances are, you probably wake up with 'sleep wrinkles' quite often, right? According to New York University professor and dermatologist Dr. Julia Tzu, you might unknowingly be adding aging lines to your face – not only on the side of your face that you usually sleep on, but also horizontal lines in your neck. What about sleeping on your stomach? Sadly, that's even worse. "The compression between the pillow and your skin can cause lines around the eye area that are more distinct than the usual lines caused by aging," she told *Marie Claire* magazine. If sleeping on your back just doesn't seem to work for you, try investing in silk sheets as well as a silk pillowcase. Your complexion will thank you for it.

Something that is gaining in popularity, however? A treatment called Bio Visage Facial Treatments. Described as a non-surgical facelift, this procedure promises near-instant toning, tightening and firming to sagging skin. "Low-level electrical impulses are used in conjunction with specialized products to improve muscle tone in the face and neck, tighten and lift jowls, soften wrinkles, and restore the glow of youthful skin...after just one treatment," explains Rouleau.

LEARN TO GIVE A PROPER MASSAGE

No, we're not talking about the neck, back and shoulders variety (although that could help too). The type of massage that French women prefer is the kind that they do on their faces. In fact, they are becoming increasingly popular in Asian countries like Japan and Korea too. Explaining the premise as a sort of "Pilates for your face", Laetitia Labassee of French skincare brand Darphin told *Marie Claire* magazine: "Aestheticians at the Darphin Paris Institute teach women to apply their face creams with a deep massaging motion." The massage she speaks of starts with applying pressure to both sides of your jawline with the pads of your hands. Gently spread the lotion further up towards the ears. Now gently apply the lotion to the apple of the cheeks, spreading up and backward in the direction of the temples. Next comes the forehead. Starting at the eyebrows, massage the moisturizer upwards toward the hairline.

PATIENCE IS A VIRTUE

In today's age of instant gratification, we have come to expect a quick-fix in all areas of our lives. The French attitude to skincare products, however? The exact opposite. The French know that the best quality products work slowly and steadily. "Skincare products can take 6-8 weeks for you to truly see results," says Rouleau. "Americans start a skincare regimen and then quickly change when they don't get immediate results." The products favored in France are much more natural, making use of essential oils and botanical extracts. "They don't use harsh and invasive ingredients that may sting and cause irritation on their skin. Many American women have the philosophy of 'if I can't feel it working, it must not be working'."

BUT SOMETIMES THE FRENCH WAY IS NOT ALWAYS BETTER...

Of course, though, nobody is perfect and that includes French women. For all their effortless grace and charm, there are some lifestyle habits that could be changed – especially when it comes to retaining the good health of the skin. Rouleau lists a few *faux pas* that French women are guilty of and how to fix them.

SUNTANNING WITHOUT SPF

One beauty practice she would advise the French population to adopt is wearing sunscreen. "Many French women still love to go to the beach and get a tan, and skiing in France certainly brings on damaging UV rays," says Rouleau. She stresses the importance of applying an SPF moisturizer to the face and neck area every day of the year, come rain or shine. "Since UV exposure from the sun (even on a cloudy, winter day) is the number one cause of aging, this isn't working in their favor."

SMOKING TO A FAULT

Dull, sallow and lackluster. Three terms you never want to be used as descriptive terms for your skin. Sadly, this is a reality for many French women who still habitually smoke. And those who don't, are still constantly surrounded by second-hand fumes in public places. According to the French Ministry of Social Affairs and Health, over one-third of French people are smokers. And even with the government introducing stricter laws and controls discouraging smoking, it remains a huge habit that has become ingrained in the culture.

Besides the myriad of dangers this poses to the rest of the body, the effects are seen mostly on the face. Smoking robs the skin cells of necessary oxygen. The result is tired-looking skin with a dull, ashen complexion. "Three years ago when I walked into a facial salon in Paris, I couldn't believe my eyes. The receptionist was smoking! Yes, actually smoking while she greeted me!" says Rouleau.

Time

Paris ne s'est pas fait en un jour!

(Paris wasn't built in a day)

There is a common phrase in France that goes "avoir la flemme". Loosely translated, this means "to be lazy". And while this may be the impression given by French women when referring to their beauty regimes, nothing could be further from the truth.

The reality is that French women prefer to spend time and effort over the weekends so that their routines during the week can be as minimalist and easy-going as possible. In her book *The French Beauty Solution: Time-Tested Secrets to Look and Feel Beautiful Inside and Out*, the founder of French skincare range Caudalie, Mathilde Thomas, shares her weekend recipe for silky, shiny hair. She mixes two beaten egg yolks with five tablespoons of rum, one-quarter cup of grape-seed oil and one-quarter cup of olive oil, and applies it to her hair. "This amazing recipe was handed down to me from my grandmother," she says. "It's not the most elegant mixture in the world, but it is very effective. It will leave your hair incredibly nourished, super shiny, silky, and with loads of body."

Modern-day French style icon Caroline de Maigret sums it up: "Nowadays, we want to be effortless. But looking effortless takes effort! So we weave a story—create an illusion of effortlessness."

And it is that illusion that has enchanted the rest of the world with its mystery. The idea is pretty straightforward: keep it as simple as possible. Have a skin condition or a beauty concern? Mother Nature has an answer for it.

In keeping with this pervasive respect for nature, French women exclusively buy their skincare products from the pharmacy - whether they have a specific skin ailment or not. The thinking behind it goes: if a product is good enough for highly sensitive skin, it has to be good for ordinary skin too. You won't find any harsh chemicals, colorants, fragrances or preservatives in them.

"Enjoy the face you have today," says de Maigret. "It's the one you'll wish you had ten years from now." De Maigret herself is a prime example of this philosophy. "I had a big nose and no boobs and apparently it was a big issue because they kept asking me to get a nose job and a boob job but I refused," she says. This is the woman who, at age 36, was asked by Chanel's Karl Lagerfeld to be the face of his St. Tropez resort fashion line in 2011.

The ultimate goal is to play to your strengths and minimize the flaws. You want to accentuate what you already have but never change anything. Hollywood may have normalized 'anti-aging" procedures like Botox, facelifts and lip injections but in France, nothing could be more unfashionable. Take Kim Kardashian, for example. For their April 2015 issue, Elle France put the reality star on their cover and it was met with huge controversy – not only from the buying public but more so from within the editorial staff. The American-born Kim does, after all, symbolize the very opposite of what French beauty holds dear: minimal effort, classic elegance and an air of mystery.

Speaking on the trends she has noticed in her own practice, French dermatologist Dr. Sylvie Bourée is succinct. She specializes in what she calls *médecin esthétique* or aesthetic medicine. French women don't necessarily want to look younger, she explains. The ideal is to remain elegant, well-groomed and, if possible, ageless.

This holistic, au naturel approach is especially apparent when you compare the beauty products in France versus the rest of the world. Globally, we are only now beginning to see an increased consciousness for eco-friendly and organic products. In France however, this has been the norm for some time. This trend towards sustainability spreads even further – not only in the composition of the skincare and beauty products themselves but also in the packaging, marketing, and shipment thereof.

One area that the global beauty industry is moving towards is technology-based skincare. Increasingly more beauty salons, for example, are steering away from manual extractions during facial appointments. These are now being replaced by ultrasonic machines that have been reported to perform the same task albeit not as harshly. This is where the French traditional template comes into play. With an emphasis on preserving the past, French beauty is slow to adapt to this technological shift. And with good reason – the French way chooses to focus on manual techniques and one-on-one consultations with individual clients. This bespoke approach relies more on the client's personal profile and the hands-on approach; something you can trust the French to pay particular attention to.

Water

Comme un poisson dans l'eau

(like a fish in water)

Hydration is something that French women take very seriously. It's not unusual to spot a one-liter bottle of water peeking out of the average French woman's handbag as she goes about her daily errands. One of the most enduring commercials on French television remains one staring ex-First Lady Carla Bruni from her earlier modeling days. Advertising Contrex water, the ex-model breezily proclaims: "Contrex, c'est mon contrat minceur", which translates in English to: "Contrex is my staying thin contract." Besides Contrex, you'll find the French supermarket shelves filled with a plethora of bottled "health water" – Evian, Perrier, Badoit, Volvic, Aix Les Bains... the list goes on.

Yes, water is big business in France, but not just the kind you ingest. The French appreciation for good old H20 extends to applying water onto the surface of the skin too. It's a common practice for women in France to refresh their faces throughout the day with some sort of facial water mist. But never the water that flows from the tap.

That's a big no-no in France. French facialists actually advise their clients against using ordinary tap water because it tends to dry the skin out.

"The base of any beauty routine is about moisture and protection," says Virginie Courtin-Clarins, the granddaughter of Jacques Cortin-Clarins, the founder of Clarins. Speaking to *The Formula Blog*, she says: "And since I love taking baths [my father] always told me that it's good to relax in a bath but never let the water get too hot or stay inside too long. He also taught me the importance of finishing with a little bit of cold water on my legs for circulation."

Through similar anecdotes passed on through the ages, the French have come to embrace the precious value of water. Sifting through their vanity closets, you'll find an arsenal of water-based products that promise more than just hydration. These are the must-have water mists to get that fresh-faced French glow:

MICELLAR WATER

It's the one holy grail product that every makeup artist swears by micellar water. Originally created as an antidote to the notoriously hard water of Paris, micellar water is essentially soft water infused with minuscule particles of oil. The tiny oil droplets are able to draw impurities away from the skin – excess oil, foundation, waterproof mascara, color-stay lipstick, the works! Wiping the skin with micellar water doesn't count as a full beauty regime in itself but as a first step before a more thorough cleanse - it doesn't get any better than micellar water.

Which micellar will work best for you? If acne is a concern for you, try *La Roche-Posay Effaclar Micellar Water* which balances oil production in the skin without clogging up the pores. *Decléor's Aroma Cleanse Soothing Micellar Water* comes with added rose oil extract, ideal for those looking for an aromatherapy experience while gently washing away surface impurities. Drier skin looking for an added dose of moisture during the initial cleanse, give *Ren's Rosa Centifolia 3-In-1 Cleansing Water* a go. Rose otto oil gives an extra pop of sweet-smelling hydration. An honorable mention has to go to *Avène Eau Thermale Micellar Lotion*. Much like their iconic Eau Thermale, their super-gentle micellar version contains the minimal number of ingredients – ideal for easily irritated, sensitive skin.

THERMAL WATER FACE MIST

According to statistics, one can of Avène Eau Thermale is sold every 20 seconds in France. That equals a whopping two million products over the space of a year! What makes it so popular? Well, unlike most other cosmetic products, it contains only one product and that's thermal water, no preservatives, fragrances or miscellaneous additives to speak of. The water is bottled right at the source in the town of Avène, where it makes its slow journey from up in the Cevennes Mountains all the way down to the Saint-Odile spring. The water collects all sorts of skin-pampering nutrients along the way such as calcium bicarbonate and magnesium as well as essential trace elements, making it ideal for sensitive and even eczema-prone skin. A favorite of not only French women,

American actress Gwyneth Paltrow is a famous fan as are British celebrities Rita Ora and Sophie Dahl.

FLORAL WATER

Nature is the French woman's biggest beauty ally – we've discovered that much. And when these botanical products smell like a bouquet of flowers, who are we to complain? Facial mists infused with flower oils are a great way to impart some much-needed moisture into your complexion and surround yourself in a haze of floral fragrance too. "In the morning I use a floral water—either rosewater or orange blossom water—followed by a mist of thermal spring water," actress Mona Walravens told Harper's Bazaar. Get your own flowery glow on with *L'Occitane Precious Mist* – a lightly fragranced mist for a quick blast of moisture when you're out and about. Another cult favorite is *Sanoflore Organic Ancient Rose Floral Water*.

MARINE MIST

We've spoken about water derived from mountains and flowers, so it only makes sense that the French would draw inspiration from the sea too. Thalgo is a brand created by André Bouclet, a pharmacist who noticed the therapeutic, healing effect that came about from the application of algae to the skin. Much like the legendary Crème de la Mer, this brand is understandably on the higher end of the price bracket due to its sought-after, difficult-to-obtain ingredients. If you are looking to spoil yourself though, *Thalgo Reviving Marine Mist* is ideal for cooling down on sticky, humid days.

BEAUTY MIST

Okay, we know something called a "Beauty Mist" is bound to draw more than a few eye rolls out there. It must be said though, *Caudalie Beauty Elixir Mist* is the real deal. Actress Liv Tyler calls it her "favorite thing in the universe"; other celebrity fans include Rosie Huntington-Whitely, Victoria Beckham and Cara Delevigne. This elixir just celebrated its 20th anniversary and is said to be inspired by Queen Isabelle of Hungary's legendary 'elixir of youth' way back in the 16th century. The mist works as a primer, a makeup setter, serum, and toner.

The Classics

Les classiques

For years, the French pharmacy was where it was at. Ask anyone in the beauty or fashion industry worth their salt what their first stop was when they visited Paris and the answer would be unanimous: "La pharmacie". It used to be somewhat of an insider's secret that the magic trick to effortless beauty could only be found in the elusive apothecaries of France. And even if you didn't understand a word of French, the only beacon you needed was the giant neon Green Cross seen on nearly every street corner. Then came the advent of the Internet and (thank goodness!) French pharmacy products could be found elsewhere in the world.

These are the most beloved must-have products that French women swear by, many of which are sold all across the world:

- The great multi-tasker: *Nuxe Huile Prodigieuse Multi-Usage Dry Oil*. Formulated with six precious oils plus vitamin E, this multi-purpose dry oil adds shine and luster to lackluster hair without weighing it down. Applied to the skin, it softens the texture, plumps up fine lines and wrinkles and moisturizes frayed cuticles.

- The classic red lip: *MAC Ruby Woo*. In fact, any of the great blue-based MAC reds will do. Russian Red is another favorite known for leaving lips with a deep, long-lasting red pigment and the added bonus of making teeth appear whiter. If red seems a bit harsh for everyday wear, take this tip from Parisian It girl Jeanne Damas. She combines *MAC Capricious* (a dark pink, near-fuchsia shade) with the much-loved bold red of Ruby Woo. "I love not using any eye makeup and putting on a vibrant lipstick," she told Vogue magazine. "I put on loads of [lip balm] to keep them hydrated. People ask me what color I'm wearing, but I mix them together, so it's not really one color." That's for during the day. For nights out, she prefers a mix of *MAC Venomous Violet, Diva* and *Viva Glam 3*. She first applies the lipstick to her fingertip and then presses the pigment onto her lips. "it really absorbs and has that melted look." To smooth out the edges and get a defined lip, she tidies up the look by going over the edges with a micellar water-dipped cotton bud.

- The hardest-working body cream: *Embryolisse Lait Crème Concentré*. Loved by American starlets Scarlett Johansson and Ariana Grande, this cult moisturizer doubles as both a primer and moisturizer and works on any part of your body – from your face all the way to your feet. Bonus: like most French skincare brands, the mild ingredients make it perfectly safe for sensitive, intolerant skin. In fact, it's been a go-to product for French makeup artists for some time. "I first spotted Embryolisse backstage at Paris Fashion Week," says the deputy editor of Vogue magazine, Lauren Murdoch-Smith. "It has been used by make-up artists for years to desensitize models' skin from continuous make-up application and removal from back-to-back catwalk shows. It then became a beauty editor secret, bought in bulk as part of the Paris pharmacy hauls during trips to the skincare capital."

- The acne-buster: *La Roche-Posay Effaclar Duo*. If acne-prone skin has been the base of your adult life long after your teenage years, you are not alone. Acne (along with the subsequent blemishes and scarring that usually follows) is a problem that is one of the biggest confidence-zappers in women. Effaclar Duo has emerged as an oil-free skin savior for its ability to target black- and whiteheads while still hydrating and improving the texture of the skin. Its texture is gel-based making it glide onto the skin for a smooth finish. In fact, French makeup artists have been known to use the wonder cream as a makeshift primer under makeup.

- The holy grail of hairsprays: *L'Oréal Elnett Satin Hairspray*. You'll know the legendary gold and white bottle if you see it and for good reason - it's a foolproof backstage staple at fashion shows the world over. Even models sing the praises of the spray. French actress and one-time face of Lancôme Alma Jodorowsky tells of being introduced to L'Oréal Elnett by her mother as a child. "My mother has eyebrows like me - she used to come at me before I went to school and tidy them," she told British Vogue. "At the time it would really piss me off but now I see it was important! All I do is spray a bit of L'Oréal Elnett Satin Hairspray onto a brow brush and brush my eyebrows with that, it fixes them - they get really messy otherwise. She wouldn't let me pluck them either, but now I am thankful."

- A lip cream for the softest lips: *Nuxe Ultra-Nourishing Lip Balm Rêve de Miel.* With its unexpected dry matte texture, another of Nuxe's signature products makes the cut. Ideal as a non-oily base underneath lipstick, it's infused with honey and natural precious oils making it a must-have in every handbag for on-the-go lip prep. "I love every product by Nuxe - all of the smells are so wonderful," says Clémence Poésy, certified French cool girl and face of the fragrance Chloé Love Story.

- The OG makeup remover: *Bioderma Sensibio H2O.* We've spoken about the French obsession of all things water-based; this product right here has to be the most iconic of them all. Bioderma micellar water can be regarded as the matriarch on which all other oil-infused water cleansers were based. It's perfectly packed with the most gentle ingredients to suit sensitive skins while still being powerful enough to tackle stubborn waterproof eye makeup. For those with dry skin, there's the Hydrabio version while oily skins will find relief in the Sébium range.

- The all-purpose wonder cream: *La Roche-Posay Cicaplast Baume B5.* Experts at targeting specific skin concerns but in the gentlest way, La Roche Posay have created this cream to target extreme skin irritation. Use it on everything from a baby's nappy rash and sunburn to dermatitis and razor burn. Then again, it's also great as just a really effective moisturizing body cream. Rough, ashy elbows? Watch them disappear after only one application.

- The no-nonsense eye cream: *Lierac Paris Diopticerne Dark Circle Correcting Cream.* Sure, you'll get fancier eye creams with lists of ingredients longer than the box of packaging. What makes this one special is that, for its relatively low price, you've got a multi-purpose under-eye cream that hydrates the delicate skin, covers your dark circles and (bonus) treats the underlying cause without being greasy or drying. The formula is filled with soothing ingredients like corn flour which truly brightens the eyes, making you look more vibrant and awake. Kind of like eye cream and concealer in one. Excellent!

- The medicinal miracle worker: *Madécassol 1% Cream.* We've spoken before about balms and lotions that soothe and calm the skin (a quality that spans across all French pharmacy brands). This one goes one step further thanks to one very unique ingredient. The 1% mentioned in its name refers to Madécassoside, a molecule derived from the Gotu Kola plant, an ancient component used in Ayurvedic medicine for years. On application to the skin, this ingredient boosts the healing process, purifies the skin, reduces inflammation, limits scarring and increases skin's elasticity. Forms of this wonder component can be found in other pharmacy products but for its purest form (perfectly safe for topical use), the 1% cream is simply magic.

- The any-age night cream: *Caudalie Resveratrol Lift Night Infusion Cream.* No matter what your age, it's never too early to start wearing a night cream to bed. And one that boosts anti-aging? Yes, please! The Caudalie brand is renowned for its breakthrough use of red wine extract to hydrate and smooth the skin thanks to an antioxidant naturally found in grapes called resveratrol. Wake up to fluffier, plumper skin and thank us later. Another Caudalie winner? Their Lip Conditioner is also worth investing in –

99.5% botanical ingredients which improve the condition of the lips over time.

• The only dry shampoo worth having: *Klorane Dry Shampoo with Oat Milk*. We know, it's not the most buzzed-about dry shampoo out there (that's a part of the allure, non?). But trust us on this one: everyone from Karl Lagerfeld to Jeanne Damas swears by this product. Comprised mainly of oat milk, this nature-infused no-nonsense dry shampoo soaks up grease on the roots like nothing we've ever seen.

From the mouths of bébés

We know... getting that French allure can be easier said than done. But don't just take our word for it. Follow these beauty tips from real-life French beauties so you too can *être canon*.

WE JUST WANT TO LOOK FRESHER, BUT THAT'S IT

"In France, we never push it," says Paris-based Dior makeup artist and Estée Lauder Global Beauty Director Violette. "We don't like to change ourselves. So when putting on makeup, we just want to look fresher, but that's it. And we like to look the same when we take it all off. You brush your brows, you curl your lashes, you put on a little bit of mascara, a little bit of blush, maybe a little bit of concealer."

IT'S ALL ABOUT BALANCE

"I like to keep my make-up pretty natural - what I choose depends on what I'm wearing," French actress Alma Jodorowsky told British *Vogue*. "If I have a long dress, something glamorous, then I won't want make-up that's too extravagant. I always try to have a balance between the make-up and the way I dress. So if I'm wearing jeans and a T-shirt I like to wear red lips to create that kind of contrast."

YOU LOOK BETTER WITHOUT MAKEUP

"A boyfriend once told me I look better without make-up, and the older I get, the more confident I am in my own skin," French model Elisa Sednaoui told *Teen Vogue* magazine. "I sometimes use a bit of kohl in the evening and I have lots of Chanel blushers. I don't use powder as I find it can make your skin look older. I don't like wearing tons of mascara so I apply a bit of brown eye shadow just at the roots of the lashes to make them look thicker. It helps open up the eyes, but no one would guess you are wearing make-up."

THREE STEPS ARE ALL YOU NEED

Lengthy, complicated skincare routines? Ain't nobody got time for that, least of all the French. Model Camille Hurel explained her simple three-step daily routine to Vogue magazine: "I cleanse with my Bioderma lotion, spray my face with rose water from Sanoflore, and then put on my cream."

THE ONE THING YOU CAN FAKE: FRECKLES

"Fake freckles—it's so cute doing tiny freckles with a brown pencil—highlights from Pat McGrath," French model Aymeline Valade told *W* magazine. "It's one thing that I do when I have to be my best, mascara, eyeliner, camouflage, and highlights done with white, shimmering eye shadow."

THE FRENCH MANICURE IS NOT FRENCH

"The French manicure is something of an enigma: it is the exact opposite of French chic. The Parisienne does not understand the point of it and never wears it," says style icon Caroline de Maigret in her book. French women wear "short, clean nails, sometimes worn with polish".

TOUSLED HAIR IS YOUR SECRET WEAPON

"Lightly tousled hair is a must to add that French touch to every beauty look," French model Joséphine Le Tutour told Vogue Paris. "I never go to the hairdresser. I am lucky not to need to buy shampoo: I am given on the shootings or in the backstages. I rarely use a hairdryer, or two minutes then I let them dry in the open air. I like it when my lengths are a little wavy".

IT'S ALL IN THE LINING

"I don't really advise an eyeliner to anybody, because you have to have your own preference," says French model Louise Follain in an interview with *Into the Gloss*. "I like pens, but crayon works for other people. My look is to do a line that begins in the middle of the lashes and very close to the lash line. Then it gets a little bit bigger and a bit pointy at the end, but not too much. It makes the eye look a bit more open".

PERFECT YOUR POUT

"A trick that I love for applying a red lip is you start with a pencil, and you put on your red lipstick, and then, you take a tissue and peel apart the two layers," French model Laetitia Casta told *Vogue Paris*. "You take only one layer and you lay it over your red lip, and then you dust loose powder through the tissue over the lipstick. It gives a nice matte finish—it's perfect."

MIX YOUR MASCARA

"I get so many tips from Tom [Pecheux, the creative makeup director of Estée Lauder]," says long-time French model Constance Jablonski, speaking to *PopSugar Australia*. "Most recently he taught me to use two different colors of mascara, black for your top lashes and brown for your bottom ones. It gives you a sharper look with more definition and makes your eyes look even sexier!"

Hair

The Hair Commandments to Get that French 'Do

"Walk into practically any office in Paris and you'll see rows upon rows of perfectly messy buns." Says Mathilde Thomas, the creator of French beauty brand Caudalie and author of the book *The French Beauty Solution*. Yes, the classic chignon may be a trademark of Frenchwoman, but that's just one in a long line of signature styles that Gallic girls have made popular.

So what's their secret? We break down the essential commandments necessary to get that effortless French hair.

THE BEDHEAD

Possibly the first thing you'll notice on a French girl? Her tousled accidentally-on-purpose bedhead, of course. We don't think it's any coincidence that Beyoncé was living in Paris when she penned those now-iconic lyrics: "I woke up like this".

The fact is, Frenchwomen probably do wake up like that, but only after putting in the necessary graft work the night before. Achieving a tousled look that's soft and textured needs constant TLC. It may look as though she just rolled out of bed but, trust us, it's all part of a bigger plan.

"Whenever possible, wash your hair in the evening rather in the morning so as not to leave the house with wet hair," says Caroline de Maigret, one of the grandes doyennes of this much-envied hairstyle.

The products you use will set the tone for the look and texture of your hair. Stay away from anything promising sleek, smooth hair. You want the exact opposite. Look for a shampoo and conditioner designed to deliver texture and a bit of volume. A volumizing mousse once you step out of the show will add some extra bounce to your locks.

"Do not dry your hair with a hairdryer (in fact, you might as well throw your hair dryer away)," says de Maigret. "Instead use two much more environmentally friendly resources: fresh air in summer and a towel in the winter." Run your fingers through your hair and spray dry shampoo onto the roots – this will stop your hair becoming oily too soon and add luscious movement to your strands.

For soft, movable curls the following morning, braid your hair into plaits and sleep in them. You'll wake up to gentle waves for that easy tousled look. Make sure the curls stay defined and textured throughout the day by spraying on a volumizing spray designed for your hair type. As the final step, set your style with a cold blast of hairspray. Your style should stay in place, ready to be shaken out and tousled whichever way you see fit.

"I always let my hair air-dry so it has a natural shape to it – every single day of the year," Jeanne Damas tells Harper's Bazaar. "While I'm putting on makeup, I keep my damp hair in a low chignon. At the end of the morning, I take out the chignon and it leaves great natural-looking waves in my hair."

Then comes the real secret of French women. "French women wash their hair less," says Australian-born, Paris-based hairstylist David Mallet. As the preferred hairdresser of French beauties Marion Cotillard and Charlotte Gainsbourg, he knows what he's talking about. "They sleep on it, not really touching it for a week, and in the end, it gets a little bit of movement and jumps around." Plus, as an extra bonus? "It also results in a lot less color fatigue and damage."

And, if you can, he recommends you switch your flat iron for your fingers. "French women actually don't tend to re-touch their hair frequently with a brush. They use their hands and massage the roots to get a lift, giving it a more organic, softer effect," he says. "Over-brushing breaks hair and leaves the ends more fragile."

BALAYAGE COLOR

"Do not dye your hair!" stresses De Maigret. "Or if you do, only in your original color to highlight it or to hide any gray." One of the greatest trends to emerge from Parisian hair salons over the last few years has been the balayage method. Favored by everyone from Jessica Alba to Kate Middleton, the coloring technique has been around since the 1970s but due to its time-consuming application, it never really caught on to the mainstream.

Cut to the present day and nearly every salon is clamoring to brush up on the sought-after technique. Literally meaning to sweep or scan, balayage differs from typical salon color in that it is applied by painting the hair strands instead of foil strips.

Remember too that, as with any artificial color added to the hair, the chemical processing can damage the fragile strands. Take special care to nourish and treat your hair regularly with oils and masques. "My own trick is to protect it with some borage oil," says Julia Restoin Roitfeld, the daughter of iconic *Vogue Paris* editor Carine Roitfeld. "It's the best nourishing oil. I also take borage as pills in the morning and put some on my skin after being exposed under the sun."

FRENCH BANGS

It's become a trademark of Frenchwomen the world over – eyelash-skimming bangs. The face that brought this style to the fashion forefront was musician and model Jane Birkin. Today, the edgy bohemian style is hotter than ever, synonymous with modern-day French beauties like Caroline de Maigret, Charlotte Gainsbourg, and Lou Doillon.

Speaking on her own signature chop, Jeanne Damas told Vogue magazine:

"Usually, I cut them myself. I like a small, unstructured fringe, which has a sixties feel, like Jane Birkin's or Françoise Hardy's or definitely Anna Karina's. Homemade and not perfect."

Then there's model Louise Follain, an almost dead ringer for Jane Birkin who captures that insouciant Birkin beauty to a tee. The Parisian It girl explained her journey into bangs in an interview with Into the Gloss:

"My skin wasn't always perfect, so when I was a teenager, I thought bangs were a good idea to hide things on my forehead... but they also made more pimples sometimes. I had them until I was 13 and then grew them out. I re-cut them myself three or four years ago. First, I wanted just to have a fringe-y bang and then it just started to get straighter and straighter. I really like Alexa Chung - she was kind of my inspiration for the cut.

"What I've learned is that it doesn't have to be perfect. If it's too straight, it doesn't work. Actually, I still cut them myself because I prefer the style to be kind of messy. The only time I go to the salon is to even the color between winter and summer."

Her foolproof technique for getting that lived-in look is dry shampoo. "If I don't wash my hair, I use Prêt-à-Powder from Bumble and Bumble, particularly on my bangs," agrees French model Louise Follain. "I think it's great because it's a dry shampoo but it also makes the hair look cool and gives an amazing texture. And you can't have oily bangs or else you look really awful."

If you're thinking of adopting French-style bags, Mallet says to just go for it. "Nearly anybody in the world can wear a fringe." A few tips though: "Most of our French clients prefer to keep [their bangs] long. It's all about the mystery," he says. Then, if you're looking to go the French DIY route, he recommends trimming your hair while dry, "without tension and without pulling on it".

Perfume

Être au parfum
(Be in the fragrance)

"For me, to go without perfume is like being stark naked," said French fashion designer Catherine Malandrino, echoing the iconic words of Coco Chanel: "A woman who doesn't wear perfume has no future".

It's this sort of vehement, all-or-nothing passion that has made the French leaders in the fragrance community. Ask any connoisseur and they'll tell you of a certain *je ne sais quoi* that differentiates every flanker of French eau de parfum from those created elsewhere. From the provocative, darkly sensual oriental notes of Yves Saint Laurent Opium to the deep flowery musk of Chanel No. 5, Gallic fragrances have always held an enigmatic mystery unlike any other.

This dedication speaks volumes to the French aesthetic of timelessness. "French women are very faithful to their perfumes. They wear the same one for years and do not change it, whether it's morning or evening, winter or summer," says style maven Inès de la Fressange to Vogue magazine. "I think American women like to have several.

They appreciate new perfumes and buy things that they discover in magazines or at department stores, where quite energetic sellers are jumping on them. This does not exist that much in France. Don't ask me about new perfumes: I generally hate them. I find them too aggressive, with too much iris, grapefruit, or I don't know what!"

Keen to infuse a spritz of French perfumery into your world? These are the unspoken rules to smelling like a French girl:

YOUR FRAGRANCE DEFINES YOU, SO CHOOSE WISELY

Dramatic as that may sound, French women take their perfumes very seriously. "The perfume builds up the other-self - the one I am and the one I wish I was," says perfumer Jean-Claude Ellena. His daughter Céline, also a perfumer, agrees. "The French woman who is extremely tailored with a lovely scarf and carries a beautiful purse— she will wear old vintage perfumes," she says. That's not to say that bold, experimental scents don't have their place. Thierry Mugler's polarizing scent Angel is one of the best-selling perfumes in France. Wear this fragrance and you may as well say: 'I love modern things, but I am seductive as well. In fact, I'm seducing you right now!' she explains.

BUT YOUR FRAGRANCE SHOULD ALSO GROW WITH YOU

It only stands to reason that the perfume you like at say, 15 years old, will adapt and mature as you grow older. "When I was a young girl, I started to wear this patchouli scent—very '70s!—until my grandfather became totally upset and told me a young girl shouldn't wear this type of heavy fragrance," says De la Fressange. "So he offered me Sandalwood by Floris instead. Later, a friend at school was wearing Chanel No. 19, and I so admired that she would have this kind of grown-up style that I copied her."

Then there is the French understanding that while love may be eternal, fleeting passions are a natural part of life. And so yes, women will have their lifelong signature perfumes but every now and then will experiment with their latest flight of fancy. "In other words, like a woman who has both a husband and a lover," laughs Ellena.

DISCRETION IS KEY

There is nothing more off-putting than having your senses bombarded with an unwelcomed fragrance. "French women do not wear very strong things," explain De la Fressange. "Perfume should be discreet, like a little secret. I spray perfume around the neck, on my wrists, and on my scarf. I guess I saw my grandmother [doing that]. She used to like perfumes so much that when I visited her at the hospital once, she only had flasks of perfumes on her table and not one medicine. It was a dainty way to receive visitors."

Then there is also the "faire la bise" - the quintessentially French greeting of three kisses on the cheeks. The idea is that you impart a subtle lingering fragrance when greeting, not an overwhelming barrage of perfume.

REMEMBER THE FRAGRANCE ETIQUETTE

While the other rules are fairly pliable, there is one massive no-no when it comes to perfume: don't ask a Frenchwoman what fragrance she is wearing. Makeup artist Laura Mercier explains the thinking behind it: "When you say, 'Oh, my God, I love your perfume,' a French woman will simply answer, 'Yes, I love it, too,'" she says. "This is because she just doesn't want to give you the details. She doesn't want you to purchase the same fragrance."

Smell like a Frenchie

So what exactly does your typical French woman smell like? If your immediate answer included the words "natural", you'd be spot on. Much like any woman around the world, scent comes down to deeply personal preference and often holds significant memories for the wearer. "I love how instant smell is - it brings you back to a place or a time incredibly quickly," says actress Clémence Poésy. "I love the smell of coffee in the morning, the smell of the sea - so many things. Basil is a smell I'm completely amazed by. And I love the smell of some people's skin, or of babies' heads."

Scent is as much a case of personal preference as it is the phase of life you're in. A teenage girl will not, for example, wear the same scent as her mother. That said, there are certain classically French perfumes that have stood the test of time and remain popular to this day. These are the most popular perfumes of all time in France:

The First Fragrance: Cacharel Anaïs Anaïs

This sheer floral fragrance is a favorite among teenage French girls. Created in 1978, this light, fresh scent is often gifted to young girls still finding their feet in the world of perfumery. With a name referencing the Persian goddess of love, this classic scent lives up to its slogan as "the most tender of all perfumes".

The Modern Parisian Scent: Chanel Coco Mademoiselle

Coco Mademoiselle was released in 2001 as a modern floral, fruity chypre and, unlike the Chanel scents before it, was specifically aimed towards the younger set. "It's the idea of a French girl. Very contemporary, chic, elegant," says renowned French perfumer Francis Kurkdjian. "The accord itself really doesn't smell like anything else you know." French actress Clémence Poésy is a big fan of this scent.

The Ultimate Classic: Chanel No. 5

The fragrance that Marilyn Monroe famously wore to bed, Chanel no. 5 is a favorite of iconic French beauties like Belle du Jour star Catherine Deneuve, Bond girl Carole Bouquet and Coco Before Chanel actress Audrey Tautou. Created in 1921, Coco Chanel's only brief to her perfumer Ernest Beaux was to craft "a woman's fragrance that smells like women . . . I want to give women an artificial fragrance. I say artificial because it will be fabricated. I want a fragrance that is composed." To this day, no. 5 remains Chanel's top-selling fragrance.

The Scent of Sophistication: Guerlain Shalimar

Dubbed as "the perfume of desire", this is often the perfume most French girls recognize as their mother or grandmother's signature perfume. "It's very, very French," says Kurkdjian. "You smell it in the theaters, you smell it at the opera." Shalimar is famously the perfume of choice for supermodel Laetitia Casta, *Rich Man Poor Man* actress Josette Banzet as well as 80s model and author Estelle Lefébure.

FASHION

Lessons in Style from the French Wardrobe

Look, we don't want to tell you what to wear. But who better than the French to impart some sartorial advice to us, lowly admirers, right? No other nation in the world is better qualified. Think of all the fashion greats – Coco Chanel, Christian Dior, Yves Saint Laurent, Jean-Paul Gaultier... yep, all French. How about we head on over to the French wardrobe for some styling tips, shall we?

MOST IMPORTANTLY, WEAR WHAT FEELS RIGHT

We all have those items of clothing that help us feel our best. Maybe it's a pair of tailored pants that cling to your hips just so, giving you a certain spring in your step. Or perhaps it's a chic blazer that makes you walk a little more upright when you slip it on. Learn to identify those shapes and colors that suit your body's natural shape. This is La Petite Anglaise blogger Ella Catliff in a fitted denim moto jacket. When choosing your own signature pieces, consider your lifestyle. You needn't invest in a tailored black blazer if smart and formal is not your style. A tailored denim piece like this one is fast-becoming a modern classic for trendy city-dwellers.

Your clothing is meant to be a reflection of who you are, after all. French women celebrate this individuality and see their wardrobes as an extension of their characters. "Stay true to your personality," adds renowned style blogger Garance Doré. "It's fun to be formal, but you still want to be able to recognize yourself."

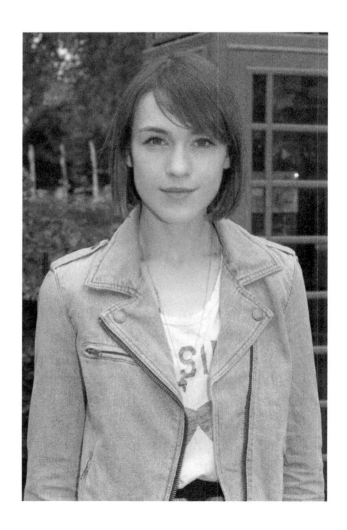

IT'S A BOY/GIRL THING

We've spoken about the French woman's affinity for all things unashamedly feminine. On the flip side, when it comes to daily street style, nothing is cooler and more avant-garde on the streets of Paris than androgynous style. Subtle nods to menswear can be seen in edgy blazers, leather ponte pants, and Doc Martin boots. Style them in your own unique way to create a standout look that's all your own – that's the French manifesto, after all. Paris-based model Anne V is the epitome of French cool in her blend of black skinny jeans, leather boots, and an edgy leather jacket.

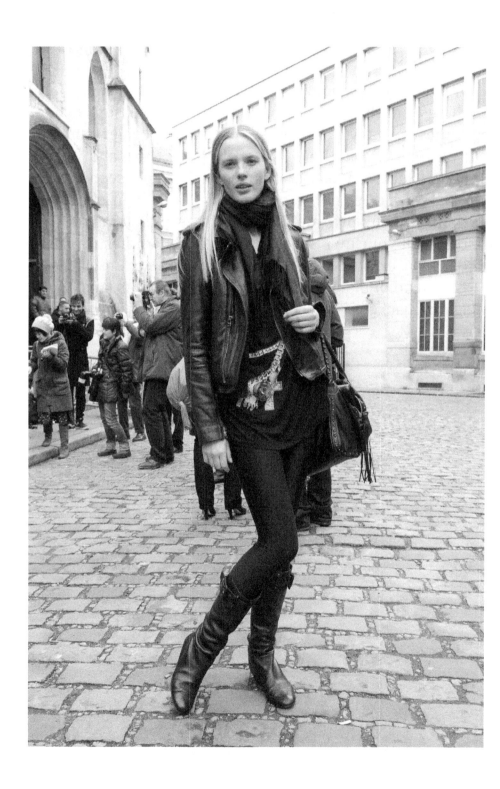

UNKEMPT GLAMOUR

We'd expect nothing less from the youngest child of Jane Birkin. An up-and-coming fashion icon in her own right, Lou Doillon's style has that sexy tousled quality that makes French glamour so hard to define. With an affinity for sheer fabrics and men's silhouettes, her fashion choices reflect the rock chic persona so fashionable today. "French-style has got to do with a certain form of arrogance, which I love," Doillon told Vogue magazine. "French girls have a tremendous respect for themselves in a way, and so they have what they want to wear, and what they won't wear—even if every magazine cover is saying, 'This is what you should be wearing'. French girls are funny like that. They have their own thing going."

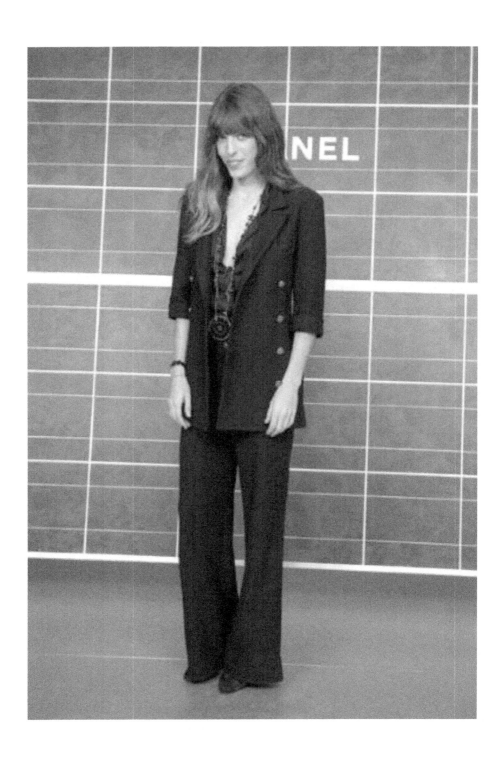

EMBRACE THE CLASSICS

Never underestimate the power of classic black and white. And when you find quality items tailored to your individual shape, hold onto them for dear life. Spotted at Paris Fashion Week, Paris-based actress Kristin Scott Thomas (considered an honorary French woman by the locals) paired the two staple colors together beautifully. In a knee-length pencil skirt and long blazer, she breaks up the color with a stark white blouse. Get her look by matching feminine makeup and hair with tailored classic pieces. Find those timeless basics that easily fit together so you've got a myriad of clothing combinations to choose from. "You don't have to spend a decade's worth of your salary on your wardrobe or flaunt designer brands the whole time," advises de Maigret. "All you need is one signature item: The one you wear when you need to feel strong."

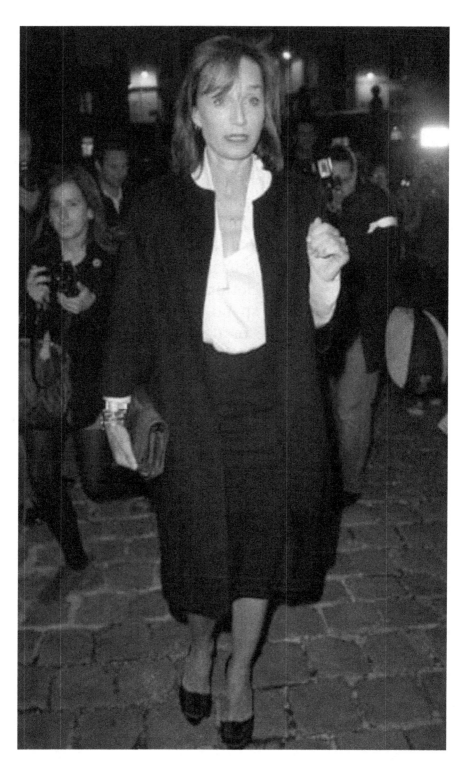

YOUR COMFORT MATTERS

In a world obsessed with fast fashion and the next best thing, it's great to find a style philosophy that embraces simplicity. Timeless French style is all about minimalism, just look at Inès de la Fressange, a former model and bona fide doyenne of French style. Her choice for all-day comfort? Wearable kitten heels or no heels at all.

"Sensuality doesn't come from heels – especially if you can't walk in them," she told The Guardian. "It's like a beautiful woman who has the perfect hair and makeup but doesn't smile. You should dress to feel good, not show off. It takes life to learn that." And she should know - de la Fressange was the first model signed to an exclusive modeling contract with the house of Chanel in the 1980s. For a dose of the former model's effortless style, remember her words of wisdom: "If you don't feel comfortable in a plunging sweater, skin-tight jeans and killer heels, go home and change".

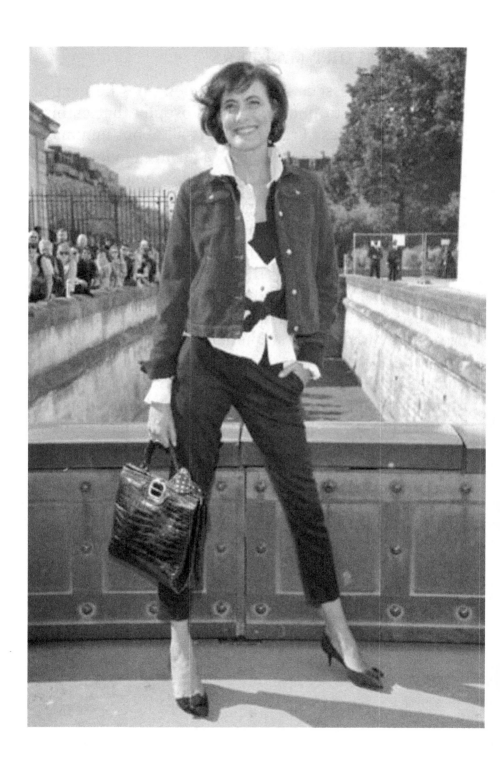

VARIETY IS OKAY TOO

The one principle that French women fully embrace is that it's okay to be who you want to be. Should that be flirty and feminine one day and moody and mysterious the next, that's perfectly fine. Legendary model and actress Laetitia Casta encapsulates this philosophy brilliantly. We've seen her in contrasting looks over the years, mixing vintage fabrics with modern accessories. She's not afraid to take risks and play with fashion, and we love her for that! Here she is in a decadently embellished tweed coat worn over a similarly textured blacktop. Extravagant, chic and oh-so French!

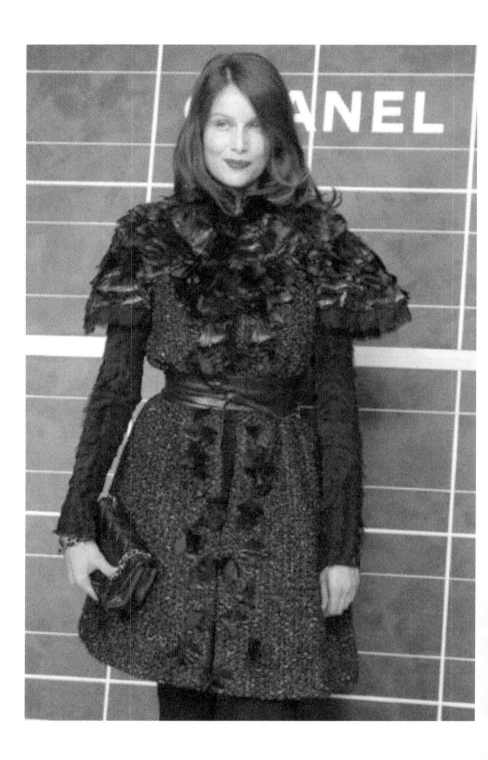

GLAMOUR IS IN THE UNEXPECTED

Who doesn't like a bit of bohemian chic? There is something sophisticated and bourgeois about throwing on an ornately patterned item of clothing and dressing it down with a pair of vintage textured boots. Model-turned-philanthropist Elisa Sednaoui is the embodiment of this laissez-faire attitude, seen here in a knee-length floral-paisley print dress and boots. Très chic!

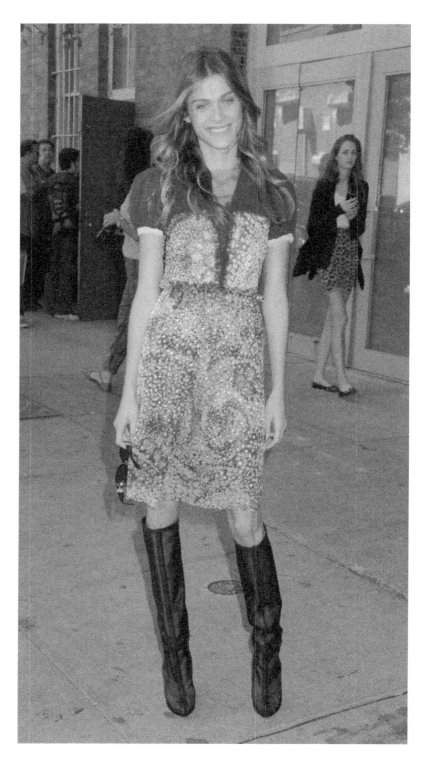

A French Sense

La vie est faite de petits bonheurs
(Life is made up of small pleasures)

Developing a French sense of style is as much about what you wear as what you don't. So what is the one thing a French woman would never wear, you ask? "Birkenstocks," says Jeanne Damas. Oh, and berets. "I do not know anyone who wears a beret," she told Vogue magazine. "The other day on a special 'Parisian-style' shoot, there was an outfit with a beret, a trench, a marinière shirt, a cigarette, and a red lip, all of this photographed in front of Notre Dame—'hardly' cliché—and we realized that nobody knew how to place the beret on my head correctly. The French stylist had to look on the Internet to check how it is supposed to be worn!"

It's this kind of outspoken you-either-have-it-or-you-don't style sensibility that seems to permeate the wardrobes of the French. For a glimpse into the modern-day clothes of everyday Parisians, we take a look at the various styles seen on the streets of Paris.

ALL BLACK EVERYTHING

If you've heard that all Parisians have a standard uniform of all black, you'd be right. The truth is that many prefer neutral shades in black and gray as a canvas to mix and match throughout the week. Where they will splash out in color is in their shoes, handbags, and accessories, as can be seen in this eclectic stylish duo spotted on the streets of Paris. This allows them to invest in quality, trend-proof investment pieces that will last beyond the current season.

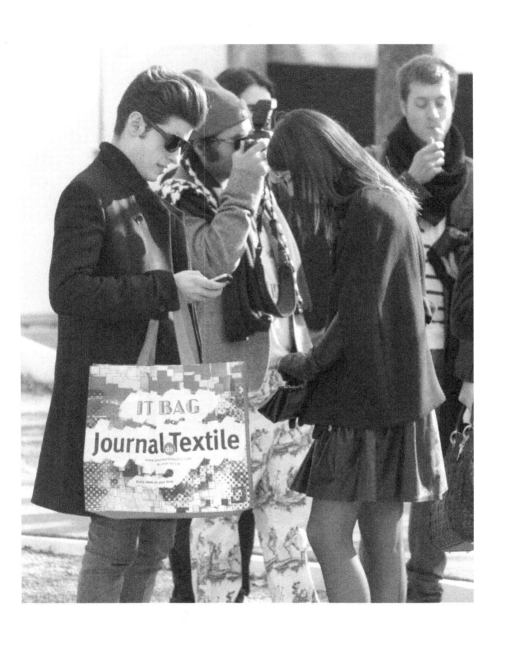

A CLASH OF PRIMARY COLORS

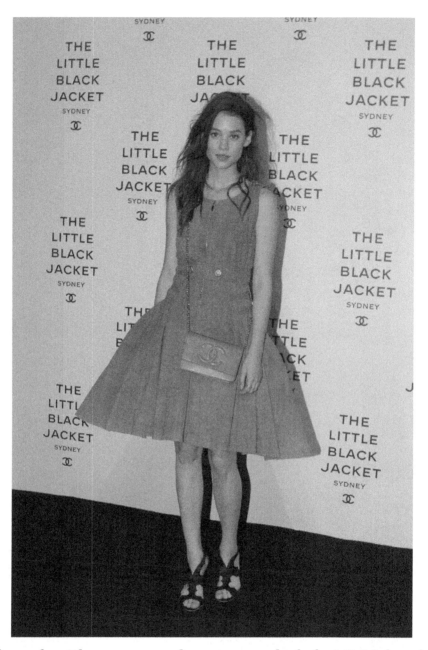

Blessed with a mane of gorgeous dark hair? Make the most of your natural olive-toned coloring and choose complementary colors like French-Spanish actress Àstrid Bergès-Frisbey. Her knee-length denim dress boasts an exaggerated A-line shape and when styled with striking red accessories, the effect is luminous.

MODERN MEETS VINTAGE

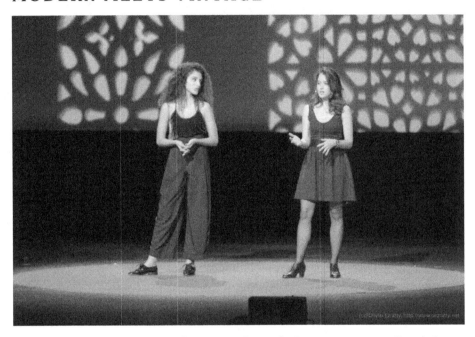

Delivering a talk at the 2015 TedxParis event, Parisians Kenza Aloui et Inès Weill-Rochant demonstrate the very French aesthetic of modern meets vintage. On the left, Kenza wears high-waisted palazzo pants, a navy blue velvet camisole top, and lace-up moccasins. Inès on the right wears a skater-style burgundy dress paired with sheer black stockings and vintage leather brogues. Their clothing choices show that, even among the youth, history is never left behind.

FAUX FUR AND STILETTOS

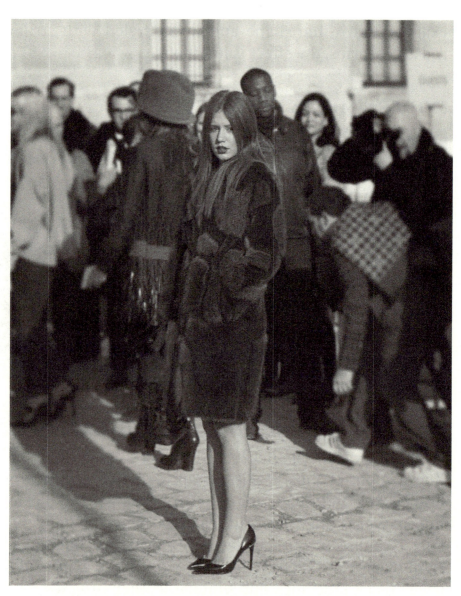

Look, it's not every day that you'll find a French woman pounding the pavement in sky-high stiletto heels – they prefer ballet flats during the day. But, for business meetings or special occasions, you can be sure that they pull out all of the stops. Here we see French actress Adèle Exarchopoulos in a stunning mix of faux fur and black patent leather heels. This outfit is unashamedly opulent – luxurious black faux fur, pointy stilettos, and bold red lips.

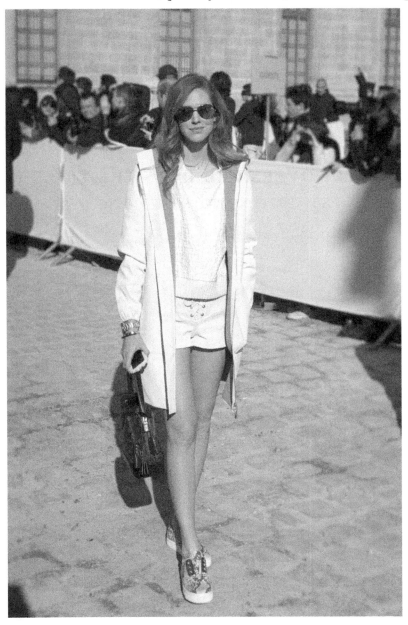

For all its insouciance of global trends, Paris is still very much a modern world city. And, like the rest of the world, the athleisure trend is highly popular among street stylers. This outfit is a prime example of urban style with a French spin. A mix of light-colored neutrals is effortlessly paired together – white shorts, a white sweater and an oversized jacket worn with metallic-trimmed snakeskin sneakers. Irreverent and cool, like only the French can.

SLIGHTLY OVERSIZED DOES THE TRICK

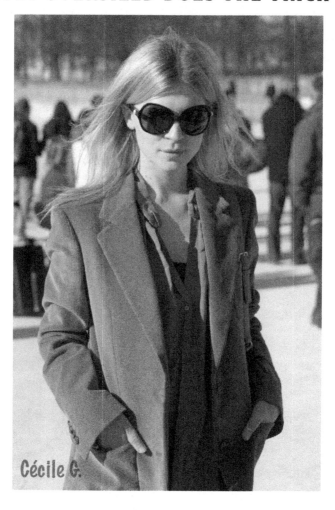

Cécile G.

We know and love Clémence Poésy for her interesting, thought-provoking film choices so it's no surprise that her street style is on point too. This look perfectly puts to rest the notion that oversized clothing can't be flattering. Here she dons a rust-colored men-style blazer just slightly too big for her petite frame. The key to wearing an oversized blazer like hers is to make sure the rest of your clothing fits close to your skin for your body to keep its feminine silhouette. An added benefit of oversized clothing? It makes your delicate body parts look slight and dainty, drawing attention to your ankles, wrists, and collarbone. "I love men's coats, especially because they're so large and they give plenty of room," agrees Jeanne Damas, speaking to Vogue magazine. "The man's coat remains one of my favorite classics."

Dressing

Être sur son 31

(Get all dressed up)

When the sun goes down, the real star power of French glamour truly gets to shine. This is when the most luxurious fabrics come out to play alongside opulent jewels and dramatic red lips. How do they manage to look so effortlessly chic at every turn? Let's take a glimpse into the stars of French cinema for a lesson in evening elegance.

COMBINE CLASSIC WHITE WITH DIAMONDS

Simplicity with a dash of elegance – that's the effect that French actress Marion Cotillard achieved in this glamorous red carpet look at the 2015 Academy Awards. The white, floor-length creation came courtesy of Christian Dior and featured an unusual eyelet pattern throughout. In sleek, sophisticated white and diamond earrings, she kept the rest of her look suitably paired down – natural, barely-there makeup and a side-swept chignon at the nape of her neck. French simplicity at its finest!

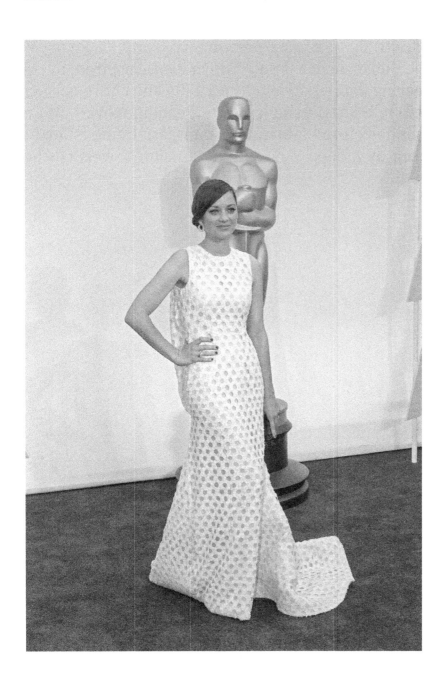

DON'T BE AFRAID OF A LITTLE SPARKLE

As one of the most recognizable faces in French cinema, actress Julie Delpy is no stranger to the glamorous nightlife. In this dazzling creation by Jenny Packham, we say she looks like a bona fide queen. Inspired by the shimmering flapper style of the 1920s, the entire garment is carefully crafted using delicate beading woven into its gauzy nude-colored fabric. Her hourglass frame is further enhanced by a deep V-neck and diamanté jewels cinched at the waist.

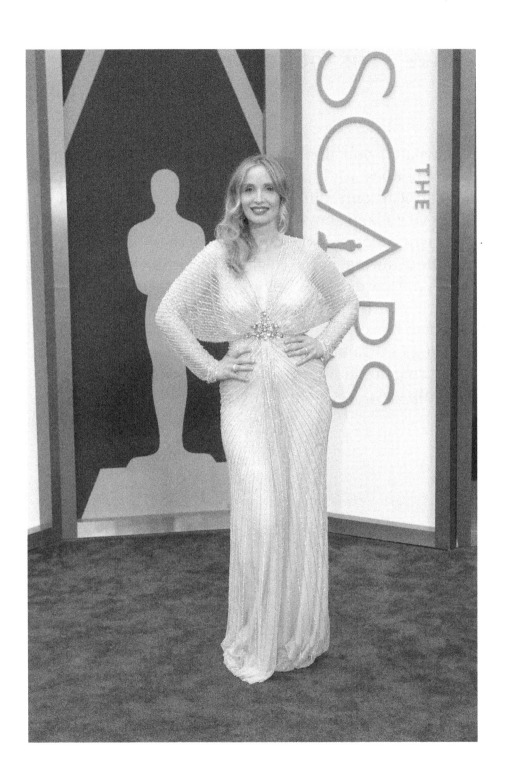

WORK WITH YOUR PROPORTIONS

So what if you don't have a so-called "perfect" body – nobody does. And, you know what? French women don't either. The only difference is that they work with what they've got and show it off to the best of their ability. Take this chic tailored look on French actress Virginie Ledoyen. Spotted during Paris Fashion Week in classic Christian Dior, her ensemble is one of form-fitting ingénue. A midi-length pencil skirt is paired beautifully with a peplum-shaped blazer. The fabric seems to mold to her body, cutting her frame at its tiniest part. This fit is particularly flattering to show off womanly curves around the bust and hip area.

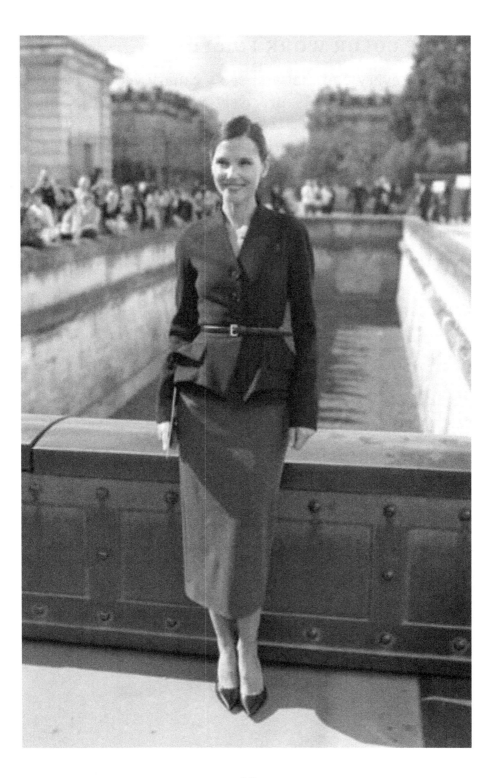

MAKE COLOR WORK FOR YOU

It's not every day that you see a canary yellow dress at a fancy event. That is precisely what makes this quirky design on French actress Ludivine Sagnier a standout winner. Snapped at the Taipei Golden Horse Film Festival, she certainly lights up the room. Is there a certain color that always gets you compliments whenever you wear it? When it comes to evening wear, a bold daring color is the perfect way to make a subtle yet unforgettable style statement.

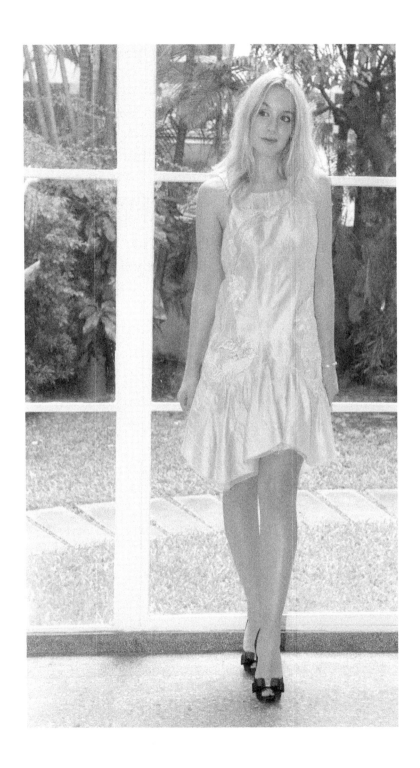

ADORN YOURSELF IN BLACK FRENCH LACE

Could anything be more typically French than sultry black lace? Renowned actress Marion Cotillard wows us again, this time in a shoulder-skimming black lace number at the Toronto Film Festival premiere of her film A Good Year. The knee-length dress is further adorned in a crisscrossed pattern over a dark gray base. To soften the dark look, her hair is loosely tied up along with smoky makeup. This ensemble is a cute, quirky alternative to the classic little black dress – ideal for a comfortable yet still elegant effect.

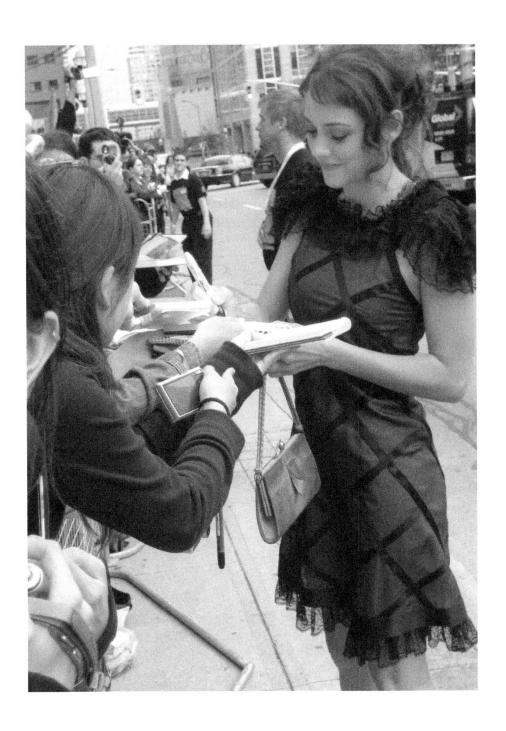

NAVY BLUE – THE SOFTER CHOICE

Black may be the classic nighttime choice but once in a while, it's good to veer away from the predictable. French politician Valérie Pécresse shows us exactly how it's done, seen here in a striking navy blue gown at the 2016 Cannes Film Festival. When selecting an evening gown in one solid color, look for one with minimal detailing and a classic, figure-enhancing shape. This navy blue design features a V-shaped neckline and a slight train - exactly the kind of elegant tailoring for understated evening glamour.

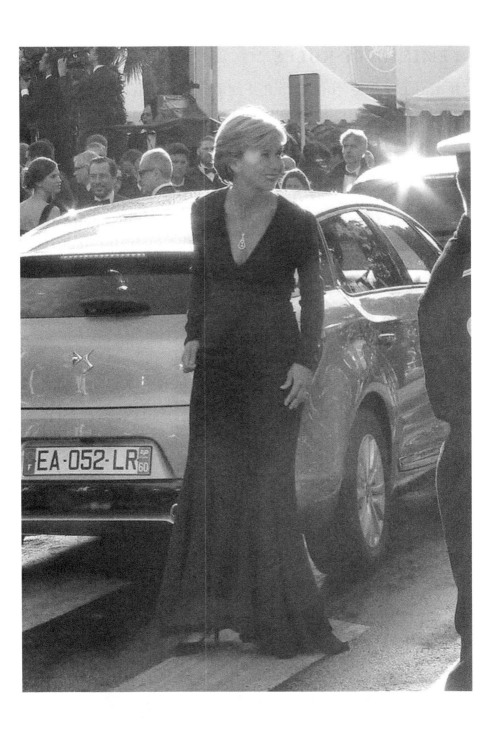

FEMININITY RULES

If there's one thing that French women love to do it's show off their fabulous femininity. Paris-born actress Élodie Yung captures a sweet yet coquettish vibe at the New York premiere of her film Gods of Egypt. She retains a sweetly innocent look despite a deep V-neckline all the way to her midriff. This look has the potential to come across as vampy and risqé, but when styled with loose-flowing locks and subtle makeup, the overall effect is soft and ultra-feminine. Un triomphe de style!

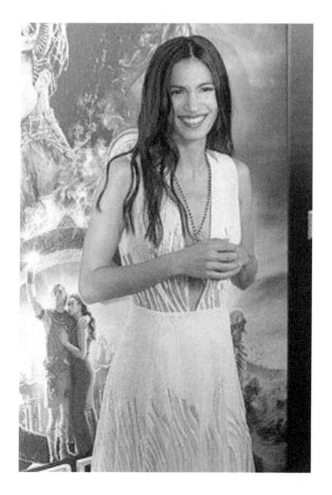

CUTE AND STILL SEXY

The age-old dilemma: you want to wear something shapely and form-fitting but still want to look classy and sophisticated. Make like Inglourius Basterds actress Mélanie Laurent and select a dress in classic white that covers your top half and shows off the legs. Featuring a mixture of fabrics and textures, this style is a shift from the usual sleek and demure evening gowns we're used to seeing. Go soft on the hair and makeup for a still approachable, relaxed persona.

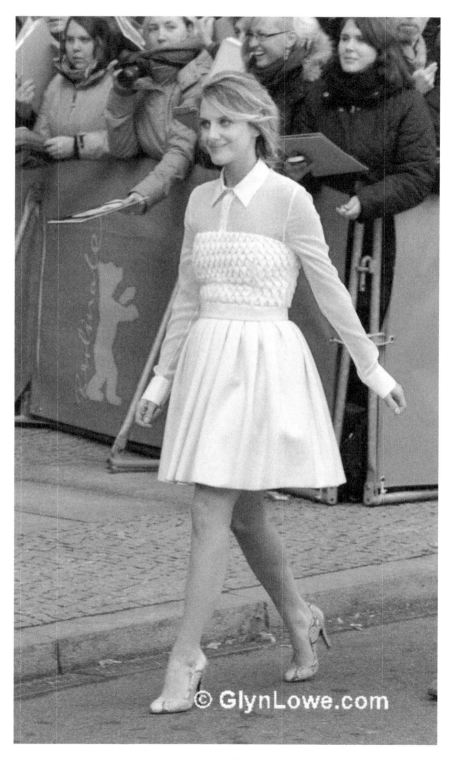

TEA LENGTH FOR UNDERSTATED GLAMOUR

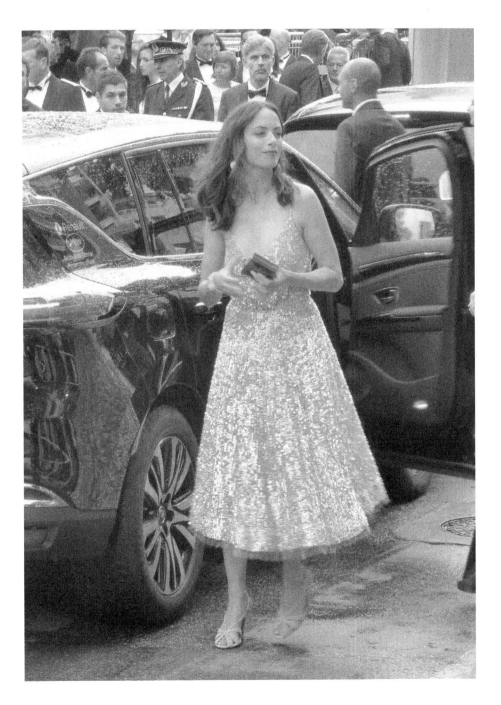

Evening wear needn't necessarily mean a floor-length gown and ultra-glamorous styling. French-Argentinean Actress Bérénice Bejo tones down her look in this shimmering dress from Valentino. A tea-length A-line style dress like this one is perfect for a cocktail event that leads into the night. To soften the look, carry the laidback feeling throughout your hair and makeup by keeping it light and natural.

IT'S OKAY TO BE A LITTLE DRAMATIC

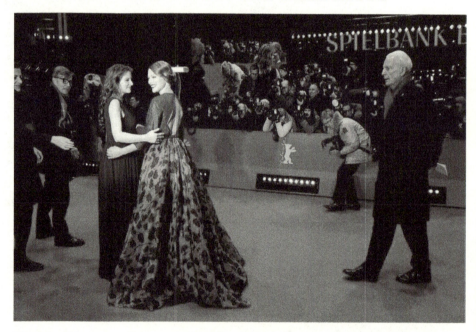

If there is one thing we've learned from French women it's that it's okay to be different. And if that means being a little dramatic and over the top, so be it! Here is French actress Léa Seydoux at the premiere of her film La Belle et la Bete at the 2014 Berlin International Film Festival. She is simply breathtaking in a statement couture gown by Prada. The decadent dress features a long-sleeved burgundy top which leads into a leaf-embossed ball gown skirt. With a matching bold lip and glossy side chignon, the effect is sophisticated and electric.

French Women

Les petits ruisseaux font les grandes rivières.
("Little streams make big rivers")

Blame it on their ridiculously glamorous Instagram snaps (you know... cobblestone pathways, quaint corner cafés, and gold-leafed street monuments), but the latest generation of French women is giving us a fair bit of Gallic envy. With effortless poise and casual cool, these are the 10 French faces *trop stylé*. Keep an eye on them... we foresee big things to come!

JEANNE DAMAS

Who she is: The quintessential Parisian girl about town, Jeanne Damas is a model, blogger, and photographer. Her latest venture is a clothing label called Rouje.

Where you might have seen her: She's modeled for big brands like Dior and H&M, but her first venture into the mainstream came through a blog she penned chronicling her daily outfits.

What makes her cool: Following Jeanne is like getting a glimpse into the real-life goings-on of the coolest girl in Paris. She takes you along to all the fashion shows, flower shops, and quaint *boulangeries* but... and perhaps best of all, on exotic holidays to places as varied as the south of France to Morocco.

Where to find her: www.instagram.com/jeannedamas

ALMA JODOROWSKY

Who she is: A French actress, singer, and model-based in Paris.

Where you might have seen her: Lancôme advertisements where she served as the brand's muse in 2015.

What makes her cool: Her husky-voiced songs with band member David Baudart are reminiscent of Jane Birkin with a splash of shiny 80s pop. Under the band moniker Les Burning Peacocks, her quirky music videos are as varied as her music's eclectic sound.

Where to find her:
www.instagram.com/almajodorowsky

FANNY PÉCHIODAT

Who she is: The brains behind My Little Paris, the first distinctly Parisian startup which curates the latest, greatest lifestyle finds in the city.

Where you might have seen her: Her company has a loyal subscriber list of four million subscribers both local and international. Are you one of them?

What makes her cool: With her two co-founders, Péchiodat launched her lifestyle company out of her living room which is currently valued at $42 million. Log on to live out all of your Francophile fantasies. In her own words: "Look like a Parisian, eat like a Parisian, dress like a Parisian, think like a Parisian—and love like a Parisian."

Where to find her: **www.mylittleparis.com**

CAMILLE ROWE

Who she is: A part-American, part-French model and Victoria's Secret Angel.

Where you might have seen her: One of the most exciting up-and-coming models today, she's modeled for Dior, Louis Vuitton, H&M and Chloé, amongst many others. In 2016, she starred in a documentary for British Vogue delving into the world of health foods and wellness. She is also the girlfriend of singer Harry Styles.

What makes her cool: Her bi-continental upbringing gives her a unique view of the world which she quirkily shares on her colorful Instagram feed. The blurb on her Instagram profile reads: "Liberté, égalité, sensualité". Nuff said.

Where to find her: **www.instagram.com/fingermonkey**

MORGANE SEZALORY

Who she is: The founder of French chic online clothing label Sézane.

Where you might have seen her: If you're an ardent eBay shopper, you've no doubt heard of Sézane. Then there's her collaboration with American label Madewell which produced the popular striped "Paris mon amour" T-shirt spotted on celebrity fans like Jamie Chung, Lily Collins and Alison Brie.

What makes her cool: Her (quite literal) rags to riches story began when she started selling vintage clothing on eBay. This foray into fashion proved an unexpectedly roaring success which resulted in the launch of her clothing label, Les Components. Seven years on, she now averages close to 20 000 orders every month – including orders from US brand J. Crew.

Where to find her:
www.instagram.com/morganesezalory

FATOU N'DIAYE

Who she is: The voice behind French beauty blog, Black Beauty Bag. Blogging since 2008, N'diaye has an impressive following of over 100 000 users on Instagram.

Where you might have seen her: Her popular website and accompanying YouTube channel, Black Beauty Bag TV.

What makes her cool: She blogs exclusively for women of color with all the scoop on the latest beauty products, trends, and innovations, not to mention snaps of her fashionable day-to-day life in Paris.

Where to find her:
www.instagram.com/blackbeautybag

ADÈLE EXARCHOPOULOS

Who she is: a French actress and model

Where you might have seen her: As one of the stars of the 2014 flick Blue Is the Warmest Color, headlining fashion campaigns for Louis Vuitton or attending glossy runway shows the world over.

What makes her cool: Then aged only 21, she became the youngest artist ever to win the coveted Palme d'Or award at the 2014 Cannes Film Festival for her portrayal in Blue Is the Warmest Color. Her Instagram feed is also peak French cool, albeit in her own modern, urban and edgy way.

Where to find her:
www.instagram.com/adeleexarchopoulos

ANNE-LAURE MAIS or ADENORAH

Who she is: Fashion editor of the hugely popular Adenorah brand since 2009.

Where you might have seen her: All over Instagram. Her feed is the picture of laidback French Riviera style.

What makes her cool: Her blogging story is the stuff that dreams are made of: Her student-run blog called Adenorah garnered the world's attention launching her prolific social media following. In her own words, she doesn't consider herself cool in the typical Parisian way. "I'm from Biarritz in the south of France – we call it French California. So my look is far more casual," she said in an interview with Topshop.

Where to find her: **www.instagram.com/adenorah**

LOUISE FOLLAIN

Who she is: A model with the Ford Modeling Agency known for her resemblance to French icon, Jane Birkin.

Where you might have seen her: At just 21 years old, she is becoming known for her street style as well as appearances at select runway shows.

What makes her cool: Not only does she look like a young Jane Birkin, she lives the same sort of fashion-forward bohemian lifestyle we've always imagined the style star to have led. Her Instagram posts are a mishmash of her cross-continental modeling journey from Paris to New York, all the way to London and back again.

Where to find her: **www.instagram.com/louisefollain**

DENNI ELIAS

Who she is: A Mexico-born, Paris-based lifestyle blogger

Where you might have seen her: Her blog Chic Muse

What makes her cool: She's a certified girl boss and owning it. As the owner of the blog Chic Muse, she's even been featured by American designer Tory Burch on her personal blog. She's also graduated with a degree from the prestigious Parsons School of Design in New York – no mean feat!

Where to find her: **www.instagram.com/dennielias**

And there you have it: everything you need to get you started on your very own voyage de style. And remember, in the words of the great Coco Chanel: "Fashion is not something that exists in dresses only. Fashion is in the sky, in the street, fashion has to do with ideas, the way we live, what is happening." À un style formidable!

One Last Thing

If you enjoyed this book, you can help me tremendously by leaving a review on Amazon. You have no idea how much this would help.

I also want to give you a chance to win a **$200.00 Amazon Gift card** as a thank-you for reading this book.

All I ask is that you give me some feedback. You can also copy/paste your *Amazon* or *Goodreads review* and this will also count.

Your opinion is super valuable to me. It will only take a minute of your time to let me know what you like and what you didn't like about this book. The hardest part is deciding how to spend the two hundred dollars! Just follow this link.

http://booksfor.review/frenchfashion

[page intentionally left blank]

Image Credits by Section

Most importantly, wear what feels right
https://www.flickr.com/photos/94941089@N03/16306558066/
https://creativecommons.org/licenses/by-sa/2.0/

It's a boy or girl thing
https://www.flickr.com/photos/51528537@N08/8533688189/
https://creativecommons.org/licenses/by/2.0/

Unkempt glamour
Photo obtained from
https://www.flickr.com/photos/myalexis/8053876365
https://creativecommons.org/licenses/by/2.0/

Embrace the classics
Photo obtained from
https://www.flickr.com/photos/myalexis/8053876365
https://creativecommons.org/licenses/by/2.0/

Embrace the classics
Photo obtained from
https://www.flickr.com/photos/myalexis/8053872369
https://creativecommons.org/licenses/by/2.0/

Your comfort matters
Photo obtained from
https://www.flickr.com/photos/myalexis/8053872885
https://creativecommons.org/licenses/by/2.0/

Variety is ok too
Photo obtained from
https://www.flickr.com/photos/myalexis/8053877624/in/album-72157631690911622/
https://creativecommons.org/licenses/by/2.0/

All black everything
Photo obtained from
https://www.flickr.com/photos/16662833@N00/4417136460/in/album-72157623572347856/
https://creativecommons.org/licenses/by-sa/2.0/

A clash of primary colors
Photo obtained from

https://www.flickr.com/photos/evarinaldiphotography/8121875672
https://creativecommons.org/licenses/by-sa/2.0/

Modern meets vintage
Photo obtained from
https://www.flickr.com/photos/tedxparis/22591082020/in/photostream/
https://creativecommons.org/licenses/by/2.0/

Faux fur and stiletos
Photo obtained from
https://www.flickr.com/photos/onepointfour/13049524374
https://creativecommons.org/licenses/by/2.0/

Athleisure a Paris
Photo obtained from
https://www.flickr.com/photos/onepointfour/13049181935/in/album-72157642129049114/
https://creativecommons.org/licenses/by/2.0/

Slightly oversized does the trick
Photo obtained from
https://www.flickr.com/photos/g-6sou/5512823201/
https://creativecommons.org/licenses/by-nd/2.0/

Combine classic with diamonds
Photo obtained from
https://www.flickr.com/photos/disneyabc/16592148776/
https://creativecommons.org/licenses/by-nd/2.0/

Don't be afraid of a little sparkle
Photo obtained from
https://www.flickr.com/photos/disneyabc/12893200874/
https://creativecommons.org/licenses/by-nd/2.0/

Work with your proportions
Photo obtained from
https://www.flickr.com/photos/myalexis/8053874232
https://creativecommons.org/licenses/by/2.0/

Make color work for you
Photo obtained from
https://www.flickr.com/photos/chiuyun/5212344704/
https://creativecommons.org/licenses/by-nd/2.0/

Adorn yourself in black french lace

Photo obtained from
https://www.flickr.com/photos/tonyshek/7025837137/
https://creativecommons.org/licenses/by-sa/2.0/

Navy Blue
Photo obtained from
https://www.flickr.com/photos/tonyshek/28076874266
https://creativecommons.org/licenses/by-sa/2.0/

Cute and Still Sexy
Photo obtained from
https://www.flickr.com/photos/glynlowe/12517303445/
https://creativecommons.org/licenses/by/2.0/

Tea length for stated glamour
Photo obtained from
https://www.flickr.com/photos/tonyshek/27501537163
https://creativecommons.org/licenses/by-sa/2.0/

It's ok to be a little dramatic
Photo obtained from
https://www.flickr.com/photos/106930755@N06/13848555803/
https://creativecommons.org/licenses/by/2.0/

Made in the USA
Las Vegas, NV
18 October 2021